Daniel Pecaut

Beating Bronchiectasis

How I Went from Diagnosis to Full Recovery in Just One Year

This book was professionally typeset on Reedsy.
Find out more at reedsy.com

Contents

Disclaimer:

I'm not a doctor.

This is not medical advice.

This book is not meant to be used to diagnose or treat medical conditions.

For the diagnosis or treatment of any medical problems, consult your own physician.

I'm merely sharing my personal experiences.

Take full responsibility for your own health.

Foreword - Dr. Michael Jung, MD

Bronchiectasis, in my professional opinion, is a less straight-forward condition to treat than most. With most other diseases, you can take a cookbook approach toward management. There's a pre-established series of steps you can take one after another. But with bronchiectasis, there's a lot we don't know and, frankly, much of the standard treatments aren't that good. Since, we, as doctors, don't know all the answers, everyone has a little different approach to treating it. On top of that, bronchiectasis is idiosyncratic in that many possible triggers and aggravating factors are specific to the individual. It's not just the negative factors that vary. What works well for one patient may not work at all for another. So each person suffering from bronchiectasis is left to experiment to find out what works best for them personally.

For this reason, I think we can all learn from each other.

I've practiced medicine for 36 years. In 1980, I received my medical degree from the University of South Dakota School of Medicine. I did my residency at the University of Iowa and was board certified in family medicine. Since then, of course, I've been re-certified in everything.

Daniel first came to me as a patient when he was in his thirties, about 20 years before his bronchiectasis diagnosis. I've seen him when he was healthy and also when he was ill. In 2012, during one of our harsh Iowa winters, Daniel was definitely trending downhill. He wasn't his normal frisky self. Although he had asthma and severe allergies, he had felt well for most of his life. With that baseline, he had an instinct for how he should feel, and that winter he knew he was no longer well.

After taking a series of antibiotics and steroids to no effect, Daniel went to Mayo Clinic to see doctors who have dedicated their careers to treating chronic lung diseases. They were able to arrest his decline, but as far as what to do next, they offered no advice except to avoid getting sick.

What's amazing about Daniel is that he did so much more than just avoid getting sick. Up until now, he had been a bystander in the process. But he could see the path he was on wasn't working anymore. His health was severely compromised and something had to change. He realized that it would be up to him to make whatever changes necessary to regain his health. He had to be the one to find the answers.

What Daniel did was uncommon. Most people are relatively passive in their healthcare. For example, I'll often ask a patient, "What medicines are you taking?" And the patient will say, "Well, I don't know. My wife gives me my medicines in the morning and I just take them."

We, as doctors, usually don't give patients all the details of what we're doing, either. To avoid over-explaining and overwhelming patients who may lack the framework to take it all in, we tend to dumb down the explanation. We instead say, "Well, this is the treatment, do this, and I'll see you next month." And most patients are fine with that.

But Daniel is one of those rare exceptions. He is bright, persistent and resourceful. He wanted to engage with the process of his own healing, so he took on the lead role in developing and leading his own recovery support team.

Daniel used all of the resources available to him to create

a customized treatment plan. He used the traditional ("allopathic") approach to medicine with treatments such as antibiotics, antihistamines, reflux medicines, and so forth. But he also realized there were more options available for recovering his energy and health than just conventional treatments, so he explored alternative approaches.

After much effort on his part, Daniel came upon the combination that worked for him. But not only that, he stuck with the regimen, day after day, in the face of much adversity. After 18 months, he went from waking up exhausted after sleeping for 14 hours to feeling rested after just eight. He regained the energy he used to have. He used to suffer from persistent stuffiness, but now his sinuses are clear. He cleared out mucus in his lungs. He increased his lung capacity so he was able to breathe deeply once again. He improved his cardio. He went from getting winded while walking to comfortably running a 10K (6.2 miles) in about an hour.

Because Daniel's story turned out so well, some people will naturally be skeptical. They will deny that his condition was as serious as it was or question whether his recovery was really as good as he described it. Nonetheless, I can confirm that he described everything accurately and honestly.

His condition, both before and after, was confirmed and documented by Mayo Clinic. I have personally gone over those records and his CAT scans. During his recovery, I saw Daniel quite regularly and monitored his health. I continue to see him today, and his overall health is undeniably better.

His outcome was uncommon, but it did happen. Bronchiectasis is a condition that can take on a life of its own. It usually doesn't get better just by good luck or the placebo effect. Normally, bronchiectasis is a condition that patients and doctors have to manage over a lifetime. I currently have two other patients with this chronic disease. Although, they started out pretty much the same way as Daniel, they're not doing as well as he is. They are struggling with flareups and other complications related to the condition.

Some people may think Daniel is claiming he's cured, but that's not the case. Although, it can be tempting to think in binary terms (black or white, good or evil, healthy or sick), that's not how most things are in the real world. We know that most conditions are on a spectrum. People aren't either well or ill. They're more in-between.

I would describe Daniel's condition as managed, in remission, or under control. But to say that his lung disease days are over would be an exaggeration. Whereas he hasn't had any issues in two years, there's the possibility that an irritation will cause his bronchiectasis to resurface. Down the road, he may need more allopathic treatments than naturopathic therapies. But as of now, the combination of what he's doing still seems to work well for him.

I wish all my patients would take such a proactive approach to their own health. That being said, some people can take that approach too far. They search the internet and try all these alternative therapies that may delay their treatment, waste their money, or, worse, make them sicker. In the medical profession, we see that all the time. Someone who has, say, type 2 diabetes will decide to treat it solely with an unconventional diet, chiropractic adjustments, or herbal supplements. In those cases, they did take their health into their own hands, but the effort was misguided, and they jeopardized their health.

When considering whether to endorse any supplement or

naturopathic treatment, my two main considerations are always 1) Is it safe? and 2) Is it effective?

The first question is relatively easy to answer. Our practice subscribes to a database where we can look up naturopathic and homeopathic treatments and get all the pros and cons of each. If it's not harmful, then I consider if it will be effective. However, efficacy is a tricky notion. Often, these treatments lack empirical evidence to support their claims. So we won't know whether a treatment is beneficial until afterwards. So it's up to the patient to try out the treatment, monitor how they feel, and decide if the treatment delivers sufficient benefit to continue.

Whenever Daniel came to me with a supplement he wanted to try, I always ran it through our pharmacy department to confirm it was safe. Then I left it up to him to decide the next step.

Daniel's treatment was safe and it appeared to be effective for him in the end. But you're going to have to be the one to decide what, if anything he did, is effective for you.

The greatest lesson of this book is that you need to take responsibility for your own health. As much as your family and medical team want you to be well, the bottom line is that you drive the process. At the same time, you should not take unnecessary risks. Always consult with your primary care physician before stopping a prescribed medication or trying alternative treatments.

When conventional medicine failed him, Daniel didn't give up. He took charge, did the research, created a medical team, consulted with that medical team, persisted despite the many obstacles, and got better. If you're in a similar situation, I encourage you to follow his example, take ownership of your recovery, and find treatments that work for you. As Daniel's story shows, that can make all the difference.

Safe journeys,
Dr. Michael Jung, MD
August 29, 2016

1

The Downward Spiral

When I was in my early fifties, I began being pummeled by frequent respiratory distress. In the winter of 2007, severe chest colds became commonplace, and a sniffle could escalate into bronchitis overnight.

In December 2011, I contracted pneumonia. I thought I had recuperated after a month or so but, over time, I started to wonder if I ever fully recovered.

The following summer, I spent a week pedaling along green cornfields with RAGBRAI (Register's Annual Great Bicycle Ride Across Iowa). While I performed well enough, I was troubled by more mucus than usual in my lungs. Something was out of order, but it hardly seemed like an emergency.

Then, in October 2012, I came down with pneumonia for the second time in less than a year. My local physician, Dr. Jung, started me on antibiotics. It didn't do a thing. He then upped the treatment to include a round of steroids, but that didn't alleviate my symptoms either.

Fortunately, I had already scheduled a visit to Mayo Clinic. When the doctor there saw my current condition, he was alarmed and called for "full-court-press medicine." I didn't know exactly what that meant, but it sounded serious. My palms started sweating and my heart beat heavily in my chest. If he was worried, I thought, my condition must be worse than I realized.

He gave me a shot of a heavy-duty steroid. "Kenalog makes people feel phenomenally better," he said. "For lifetime asthmatics, it's often the healthiest they have ever felt."

Unfortunately, like previous treatments, the Kenalog didn't do a damn thing for me.

That stunned and puzzled him. He said he'd never had that happen before.

My condition continued to deteriorate. Through December 2012, my body was weak from the strain on my lungs. Doctors kept throwing medicine after medicine at me. I took each one, thinking surely that something would work, but absolutely nothing had any effect.

I was in free fall with no parachute. My lungs had lost their resilience, and I was losing hope. My health continued to get worse. I called Dr. Jung and I told him my lungs were not rebounding. He prescribed ten days of Levaquin, a deep penetrating antibiotic with a high risk of side effects like nausea, vomiting, insomnia, and abdominal pain.

Too weak to drive myself, I had to wait for my wife, Kay, to pick up the prescription while she was taking care of some last-minute Christmas shopping. Contending with the rush and frenzy of the holiday season, she weaved through the crowds and traffic as fast as she could. As I sat at home waiting for her, I could feel myself slipping — almost melting away. For the first time in my life, I thought, *Maybe I'm dying*. When she finally burst through the door, at about 4 p.m., I grabbed a glass of water, popped open the bottle and immediately swallowed the tablets.

That night, I feared I might not make it. Would I have to be rushed to the hospital? Would I even wake up again? I slept upright that night — fighting for every single gurgling and labored breath. That focus, in a way, became a form of meditation, though I certainly wasn't thinking of it that way at the time. It was the bleakest night of my life, filled with endless anxiety and a fear that I would never see the morning.

But I made it.

When I awoke to daylight coming through my window, I was still very weak but I felt slightly better. I could breathe a little easier, but I wheezed like a 90-year-old man. I could barely shuffle from my bedroom to the kitchen.

There's a state that I learned about through my Zen training. You can enter *samadhi* after a long meditation. In Sanskrit, it means "unreasonable joy." That was the state I was in. Everything seemed clearer, brighter, and more beautiful. My heart was open. I felt so much love from Kay and my children. I was grateful. Everything was electric. Every emotion was magnified. My cinnamon raisin bagel tasted divine. I was still a mess physically, but spiritually I had never felt more alive and joyful.

I was running out of treatment options, so I was grateful that the Levaquin had worked. It was the bungee cord that had pulled me back from a free fall.

Even though it seemed I was on the mend, I felt like a shell of who I once was. Still full of mucus, I fought for every breath. I didn't want to go downstairs because I was afraid I wouldn't be able to climb back up again.

That Christmas, I saw the concern in my kids' eyes. Rather than sugarcoating and trying to reassure them, I decided to play it straight. I told them I had almost died and that I was still very weak. I had no strength. I was scared of getting sick again. This experience had destroyed my expected pattern of illness and recovery.

It took until April 2013 before I was well enough to return to Mayo to find out what happened. When I arrived, the staff marveled at my condition. Apparently, I was an interesting case, and I appreciated the attention.

Mayo Clinic's diagnostics are top-notch. They took cultures and ran a variety of pulmonary and lung function tests on me over a six-week period. I was grateful for their thoroughness and process of elimination.

They were positive they were going to find a virulent tuberculosis-related strain called mycobacterium avium complex (MAC). MAC is, apparently, very difficult to get rid of. My doctor said he has patients who take one antibiotic for six weeks, then another one for six more weeks, then switch to a third type for six more weeks, and so on. This rolling protocol was so that the strain would not become resistant to any one of these heavy-duty antibiotics. I remember thinking, *Jesus, I don't want to do that.* It sounded awful.

When all was said and done, the final diagnosis was bronchiectasis. This is a chronic condition where airways become inflamed and scarred, usually as a result of an infection. The doctors said I most likely had permanent lung damage.

If I got sick again, it would restart the same downward spiral. The damaged lungs would retain mucus again and create a high risk of infection. This infection would make me sick again, which would cause more damage. The damage would increase the likelihood of more infections.

As I left, I asked, "So, what do I do now?" They replied, "Don't get sick."

I was incredulous. *Really, that's all you got?* But I appreciated their directness and honesty. There was no dancing around it. They said to avoid airplanes and crowded theaters. "Be aware that getting sick is what will exacerbate your problems. If you don't get sick, then the rest of the spiral cannot happen."

I didn't like the sound of that at all. The most knowledgeable experts in the country had just said there was nothing more they could do. My best option was to quarantine myself from society. The healthcare system I had always trusted essentially told me, "We've done all we can for you. From here on, you're on your own."

2

How This Began (or Five Decades of Health Issues)

In a panic, I kept repeating to myself, "I can't breathe. I can't breathe, I can't breathe!"

Gasping for breath, I felt like there was a plastic bag over my head. I didn't know what was happening to me. I looked at my parents for support, but they seemed as terrified as I was.

Minutes before, my family and I were having a relaxing Sunday afternoon swim at the Sioux City Boat Club. Now everything was collapsing.

Somehow my parents got me into the car and drove me home. I don't know why they took me there instead of the hospital.

My field of vision collapsed as we entered my bedroom. Lying in the fetal position, all I could see was the orange and black carpet at the bottom of my bookcase. I could hear their frantic voices as they made calls, reaching out to anyone who could help. Although my parents were close by, I felt alone.

Slowly, I began to notice I could breathe a little deeper by calming myself. Although I didn't have the words for it yet, I was learning to detach—to let go and passively observe my thoughts, feelings, beliefs, and emotions. The message became clear: I'm all alone, and I have to go within in order to survive.

Then my dad's friend, who was a doctor, arrived at our house. After quickly examining me, he gave me an inhaler — my first of many. It opened up my lungs immediately. Things calmed, and I was alright for the moment.

That was when my respiratory issues began. I was five years old. As if that wasn't bad enough, shortly afterward I also started developing a variety of airborne and food allergies.

Peanuts are my worst allergy by far. They lead to an anaphylactic reaction.[1] Over the years, I've had many accidental exposures to peanuts that could have killed me. It's just something that would happen once in a while. Something would slip through the radar, and then I would be in a horrible situation.

For example, a friend's grandmother once assured me that the nuts in her "famous brownies" were walnuts, which were fine for me. It took only one bite to know they weren't walnuts. They were, of all things, walnut-flavored peanuts.

The response was immediate. I felt severe nausea, my mouth filled with saliva, and my throat tightened. I had essentially

---

[1] The Mayo Clinic's website defines 'anaphylaxis' as the following:

"Anaphylaxis is a severe, potentially life-threatening allergic reaction. It can occur within seconds or minutes of exposure to something you're allergic to, such as a peanut or the venom from a bee sting.

The flood of chemicals released by your immune system during anaphylaxis can cause you to go into shock; your blood pressure drops suddenly and your airways narrow, blocking normal breathing. Signs and symptoms of anaphylaxis include a rapid, weak pulse, a skin rash, and nausea and vomiting. Common triggers of anaphylaxis include certain foods, some medications, insect venom and latex.

Anaphylaxis requires an immediate trip to the emergency department and an injection of epinephrine. If anaphylaxis isn't treated right away, it can lead to unconsciousness or even death."

been poisoned, and my body was trying to rid itself of that poison.

When I first started having these reactions, I feared every time would be fatal. I quickly learned to make sure I always knew how to get to a hospital.

Because of my various health issues, it felt normal to go to the doctor on a regular basis. Doctors seemed like gods to me. They were always bigger. In their white coats and with their bright examination rooms, they had an imposing presence. With his low voice, my family physician even sounded like God. I had total trust in him. He seemed infallible. Whatever he said, that's what I would do — no questions asked. It wasn't until I grew older that I found out my mom had a grudge against him. She developed this grudge precisely because he was fallible.

As a child, I had a lot of problems with fluid in my ears. Because of the fluid, my earwax began to harden. He said it was okay, but my mom didn't believe him. Following her instincts, she took me to another doctor for a second opinion.

The second doctor told her, "We need to do emergency surgery and get that wax out of there or he'll lose his hearing entirely."

I needed to have a myringotomy, which would put a hole in my eardrum so a little blue tube could equalize pressure from both sides. That procedure was fairly new and just one doctor in the area specialized in it: Dr. Donaldson. My mom and I flew to Iowa City to have it done.

My older brother and two younger sisters were jealous because I got mom to myself. At home, my siblings and I competed for her attention. I normally didn't get much of it because I was quiet and shy. My siblings did most of the talking while I just listened.

That trip was a big deal for another reason. As a child, I somehow got the notion that I wasn't wanted. So, every decision I made was to avoid rejection or even mild friction.

For all my issues, I had a nice childhood. I was born and raised in Iowa. I grew up in a brick house in an upper-class neighborhood with tree-lined streets. My father owned Pecaut & Company, an investment business that he, my grandfather, and uncle had founded together. My mom was active in the Episcopal Church and community volunteering.

I was timid. What I wanted most was safety. I'm not quite sure why, but I wasn't a risk-taker. I removed uncertainty whenever I could. I needed control. I never jumped into the water unless I had first checked its depth and temperature. When faced with two possible routes, I always took the safer one.

I deliberately constructed a safe environment. I was hyper-aware of possible threats, so I avoided things. I just stayed away. I was once bit by a dog. After that, if a buddy of mine had a dog, he could come over to my house and play, but I wouldn't go to his.

I was shy. My drive to go outside wasn't as strong as it was for other kids. I loved to read, almost to the point where my parents had to kick me out of the house to go play. On a Saturday, if I had a good book to read, I was happy. I didn't feel like I was missing out.

I felt somewhat frail, but that didn't slow me down much. I played less-than-full-contact team sports like church basketball, touch football, and Little League baseball.

Then, in high school, for reasons I still don't understand, I temporarily outgrew my health issues. I ran on the cross-country team all four years. I was always in the back of the pack, but I was excited to be part of the team. I liked the esprit de corps of everyone doing the same hard workouts. On the last day of the cross-country season of my senior year, I clocked a five-minute mile. That was my best time ever. What I didn't know was that I was in better shape that day than I'd ever be for the rest of my life.

While attending Harvard that fall, my allergies returned and I developed "athletic asthma." Whenever I ran, I'd get wheezy. One day I went for a run but had to stop a mile from home and walk back because I just couldn't go on.

My family liked the idea of me coming back to Iowa to work in the family business. So after I graduated, with the class of 1979, I moved back and went to work for my father.

During summers in high school, I had worked there part-time in the back office. I did grunt work, such as filing S&P 500 tear sheets that had to be alphabetized in color-coded encyclopedia-like binders.

When I entered the firm as a full-time employee, I felt inadequate. I graduated with a degree in philosophy and had no clue what I was doing or what was going on. Our small family-run operation didn't have a formal training program. I felt isolated. I tortured myself with self-judgment and doubt. I tried to learn by showing up and paying attention. There was a lot of trial and error.

I married my high school sweetheart, Kay, when I was 22. At age 26, I became a father when Kay gave birth to our first son, John.

By then, I was thinking about moving to a major city to work for a big financial firm. But I chose the safer road of staying at home, at the family business.

At age 28, my father and I bought out our partners, and I became an owner at Pecaut & Company. I was a workaholic. I liked being busy because it was something I could control. I knew that if I worked hard, I'd get better at my job. Working late was also a way to avoid my wife when things weren't going well at home.

As I grew older, my body's biochemistry continued to change. I was now reacting to more foods than ever. Apples and peaches now caused allergies. My reactions to watermelon, celery, and carrots worsened. As time went on, it took less and less to trigger a wheezing spell. As my body rebelled more and more, I worried that soon I would be able to consume only water and toast. There was definitely reason for concern.

Thankfully, I had a college roommate, Rick Kvam, who worked at Mayo Clinic in Rochester, MN.

As far as the medical establishment goes, Mayo is the mecca of traditional healthcare. Universally acclaimed, it is the best conventional medicine has to offer.

When I told him about my latest health situation, he suggested that I come up to the clinic to get checked out. I met with a Mayo allergy specialist in late 1985.

I told him about my allergy to potatoes. "If I peel them, I'll start sneezing."

He laughed and said, "Potatoes are like 98% water."

He followed up, "If you eat French fries, do they bother you?"

I told him they didn't.

He tested me for allergies by putting a small amount of different potential allergens under my skin, up and down my arm. After a few minutes, he said, "You reacted to almost everything we tested you for. You're one of the most sensitive people I've ever come across."

He was pretty nonchalant about the allergies. His prescription was simple: "You are your own best guide. If something bothers you, don't eat it. Once in a while, you can try a tiny sample of something you've had reactions to in the past to see if you still react. That's the best you can do."

However, he was alarmed by my lung capacity, which was half of what a man my age should have. I had always wheezed, but I was active and felt okay. He told me that if my lung capacity declined much more, it would impede my ability to do things and probably shorten my life.

He prescribed a corticosteroid inhaler, which had recently been introduced as a therapy for asthmatics. The device put steroids into patients' lungs to temporarily suppress their immune system so their body wouldn't over-respond to allergens and cause an asthma attack. I took a few puffs of this a day. I was also given Ventolin, an albuterol inhaler, for emergencies. Ventolin opens up the airways of constricted lungs. With that one-two punch, the doctor felt that I should be able to manage just fine.

What I didn't know at the time was that the prolonged use of corticosteroid inhalers could lead to a failure of a person's immune system. That put me at risk for being knocked down by some biological agent. Like kryptonite, something that wouldn't bother most other people could wreak havoc on my body.

Back then, the long-term consequences of corticosteroid inhalers weren't well understood. Now I see that I had been regularly (and purposefully) suppressing my immune system for 30 years.

I was at risk without even knowing it.

3

Coming to Terms with the Diagnosis

After Mayo gave me the diagnosis of bronchiectasis in April 2013, I was so shocked that I didn't have much discussion with the doctors about what the condition was.[2] I had to do my own research to learn more.

What I found overwhelmed me. There was so much information out there. Yet, at the same time, this condition is not exactly mainstream. There weren't any real books about it on Amazon.[3] It's a bit on the fringes. So I searched. And the more I read, the worse it sounded.

I looked at online groups of bronchiectasis sufferers. One woman said she was coughing up blood. Another had to have a lung removed because the damaged areas, if left in, would create more problems.

None of my close friends had ever heard of the condition. Even though I'd been a respiratory sufferer all my life, I had

---

[2] Leaving with a lack of information is a devastatingly common occurrence. I would later read about people who were simply given a pamphlet. One woman's doctor wrote "bronchiectasis" on a napkin and was told to go home and Google it.

[3] There still aren't.

never heard the word until that day at Mayo. It seemed as if I was in a small group.

After some research, I found that most people who get bronchiectasis have HIV or tuberculosis. That was strange and confusing. I wondered, *How did I get in this group?* Then I realized our commonality: our immune systems are suppressed. I struggled with feelings of anger and confusion. I thought, *I don't belong in that group. How unfair!*

To be honest, I still don't quite understand bronchiectasis. But here's what I do know about it:

- When airways are damaged, the lungs can't expel mucus like it should.
- Excess mucus creates an environment for infections to flourish.
- When that happens, you get sick.
- When you're sick with a respiratory ailment, more lung tissues get damaged.
- That increases the size of the hotbed where mucus doesn't flow properly, which makes you more likely to get sick again.
- As the damaged area gets bigger and bigger, the lungs are less and less able to expel mucus.

It's a vicious cycle. Eventually, the only way to try to stop the system's deterioration is to remove part of the lung. It's like amputating a gangrenous body part, and the surgery doesn't always work.

The more I read of bronchiectasis sufferers' stories, the less I wanted to be part of this group. But I was in that group.

My life was in danger, and I needed to do something about it. I just couldn't accept my fate. I was intellectually aware that the diagnosis was real, yet I was still in denial. I felt healthy enough to delude myself into thinking I could *choose* not to have this outcome. In the back of my mind, I wondered if the Mayo doctors got it all wrong. I was resisting.

I shared details of my diagnosis with my business partner, Corey. The rest of the staff got a brief overview. I didn't talk to clients about it. Beyond my small inner circle, I didn't discuss it with anyone. I kept my condition private.

I struggled intensely on the inside. Even with Kay, I didn't share the full depth of my terror and grief. I wanted to protect her, not scare her. I shared enough, but I was careful not to overdo it.

It wasn't just death I feared. I feared losing control of my life, losing my ability to function, and living in pain. I feared being alive yet not living well. I dreaded the water torture of a messy decline that could go on for another twenty years — a decline that would include frequent doctor visits, having parts of my lungs removed, and reduced capacities. I was terrified by the thought of constantly struggling for breath and not being able to move around. I didn't want to go back to that dark night in December 2012, but I could easily end up there again. That could be my entire life. The life I knew and loved could erode away.

My brother, David, died of lung cancer in 2009. He was hooked up to a breathing machine, fighting for every breath. It was painful to see him suffer. I didn't want to suffer like he did.

My mother became a deacon at age 65. Then, within a matter of months, she was diagnosed with terminal cancer and was dead by the next year. She had finally heard her calling, and then she died.

David had a similar experience. He was at the pinnacle of his powers as a networker and social entrepreneur. Influential people wanted him to run for mayor of Toronto. He was considering it, and then his life was over.

They both had the experience of arriving at exactly where they wanted to be, only to have death and disease snatch it away. Because of this, I had the belief that when you get to the peak of what you're able to do, you die.

At the point of my diagnosis, I was riding high on a streak of successes and achievements. Under my leadership, the investment firm was thriving. The regional Goodwill branch, of which I was a board member, had just built a $2.5 million community center. I was also instrumental in saving a personal development organization that changed my life: the ManKind Project. All these achievements happened at roughly the same time.

I felt as if I was finally able to realize my vision and make things happen. Also, this period marked a high point in my marriage.

So, this must be my time to die.

4

Getting Clear

Deep in denial and despair, I was lost. I didn't know where I was going. I needed help and direction.

Jun Po Roshi, who had offered me counsel for years, provided that help. He is the head of the Hollow Bones Mondo Zen Order. He's a direct descendent, the 183rd patriarch, in the Rinzai Zen tradition.

Jun Po issued me an invitation. He was going to be leading a special seven-day silent meditation retreat in upstate New York that June. The venue, Dai Bosatsu, is the largest Zen monastery outside of Japan. Although Dai Bosatsu is the home base of the Hollow Bones Order, it was the first time Jun Po had returned since he trained there as a monk. In a falling out with that community, he had left. Now, after 20 years, those wounds had healed. Jun Po had reached out, and those at the monastery decided it was time for him to return. It was going to be an emotional and special event.

I told Jun Po that, while grateful, I couldn't go. I was too tired and sick.

I appreciated his direct but nurturing side in that moment. He said, "We'll take care of you. If, at any time, you need to sleep, go to bed. But you need to come."

In June 2013, I flew to upstate New York.

Arriving there, I was amazed by the spectacular Japanese architecture of the monastery on a beautiful mountain lake.

True to his word, Jun Po looked out for me. At about 6 p.m. on the first day, I felt exhausted but didn't want to stop. I'm wired to not quit, no matter the difficulty or the cost. He looked at me and, in a fierce warrior-like tone, said, "Go to bed — now! I'll see you tomorrow." I went to bed and passed out immediately. I slept for twelve straight hours.

Feeling safe and supported created the space necessary for me to do the work to come.

My second day at Dai Bosatsu was pure grief.

At its deepest level, the training of Zen meditation is to not look away. The idea is that all of our neuroses and pathological behaviors are forms of turning away from reality. In Zen, it's painfully simple: We sit on a cushion with our eyes open, and we breathe. Breath after breath. Whatever arises, arises. We sit and don't move, no matter what. The training is to stay with it.

At this retreat, we would sit hour after hour, day after day, in this state.

For all my denial, I still believed in healthy process and practice. In my mediation process, I don't get clear every day, but, over time, I trust that the clarity I need will emerge. I just need to stick with it.

I trusted in this process, no matter how painful it was. I knew it was healthy and necessary to go through. So I sat. I didn't move. I didn't look away. I must have looked like a mess, with snot running out of my nose and tears streaming down my cheeks. But I wasn't going to turn or look away. I was going to stay right with this and process it.

In that state, I could not — would not — run from life. In that silence, all my grief arose. I was grieving my impending death. I was grieving the loss of my wife, my children, my friends, and my entire life. I was absorbed by how much I loved Kay. I didn't want to leave her. I loved my children. I didn't want to leave them. I loved my life. I loved my friends.

Life is impermanent. It's all temporary.[4] Yet I was still so attached to it.[5]

I had to grieve my own death. That had to happen. I had to pass through the grief to go beyond it. At Dai Bosatsu, I was grieving my own death at a level I could not have touched otherwise.

Also at that event was a Zen priest named Suzanne Friedman. She had had cancer. She had dealt with it with meditation, Qigong[6], natural herbs, and so on. It had gone into remission. Recently, the lung cancer came back, so she was up against it again.

Jun Po made a point for Suzanne and me to get together and chat. It was a silent retreat, but my situation was so severe that

---

[4] The first great truth from the Buddha is impermanence. Everything is impermanent. Everything is on fire. Everything dies.

[5] The second great truth is about suffering. Suffering comes from the stories we tell about ourselves and the attachments we make to that which isn't permanent. When we choose to, we can let those go, and the suffering stops. Or we can continue to hang on, and the suffering continues. Life has pain, but suffering is optional.

[6] A meditative physical exercise similar to Tai-Chi.

Jun Po made an exception for us. We talked about her story. It was so powerful to see that she was there, in her own struggle, modeling a healthier way of living.[7]

On the third day came a turning point.

While sitting perfectly still in meditation, with tears running down my face and snot coming out of my nose, it happened.

My brother-in-law, Youssouf, had told me this traditional Mauritanian story years ago, and, out of nowhere, it popped into my mind:

> *Joha is the village simpleton. While he is sleeping one night, burglars sneak into his hut and steal everything, including the cot with Joha on it. As they are going down the street, they hit a bump and Joha falls off the cot. He wakes up, sees what's happening, and starts dancing and singing. He's so loud that he wakes up the neighbors. They ask, "Oh, Joha. What are you doing? People are stealing everything, and you are dancing and singing. Are you crazy?" Joha responds, "I just can't wait to see where we're moving to."*

As I sat with this story, I wondered, *What was that about? Where did that come from?* I didn't understand it.

Then it hit me: Joha is me. I'm in the same situation. Robbers had come and stolen the life I knew. I can either go on grasping and clinging to what I've lost, or dance and sing on my way to

---

[7] She passed away in 2014. Before she died, she wrote a beautiful book called *Zen Cancer Wisdom*. She starts each section with a quote from a Zen master, explores what it means, and then applies it to daily living. She was beautiful, amazing, and courageous.

what could be. I could open myself up to where I was moving.

It was a profound realization. I didn't snap out of my grief, but the story gave me total clarity. I saw an opportunity. I had a choice as to how to deal with my life as it was.

That was the turning point. I declared I would dance and sing. I wouldn't cling to the past and the way things were. I would let go, accept reality, and ask what my life was going to look like now. It meant engaging rather than passively accepting my fate.

I finally accepted. *I am dying. I need to do something about it. This is serious.*

Life isn't permanent. We all have a death sentence. But that doesn't mean I should accept any death sentence with open arms. I will die, but it doesn't have to be here, and it doesn't have to be now.

Since conventional medicine couldn't help me, I resolved to dive into integrated medicine and find out what was there. What exactly "integrated medicine" meant or how it would unfold, I didn't know, but it was time to learn.

There was an adventure waiting for me. This time, I was not going to take the safe, established route. The stakes were too high. I needed to do something out of the norm, or I would die a slow death.

So I stepped away from the system I had always known and stopped thinking the way I had always thought. I opened my mind to new possibilities.

I came back from that retreat reinvigorated, with a new perspective. I came back home clear.

5

Assembling the Team and Making the Plan

Even though I had my breakthrough at the retreat, I didn't actually know anything about alternative medicine. The breakthrough told me just where to look and how to be open. I still needed knowledgeable allies to show me the way.

I was raised to value rugged individualism, lone rangers, and pulling myself up by my bootstraps. But that leads to living in isolation, particularly around things that matter.

In 2003, ten years prior to my bronchiectasis diagnosis, I started shifting how I operated in life.

I joined an international personal development organization, the ManKind Project (MKP). Thirty years ago, its founders looked at the feminist movement and wondered why men weren't redefining their roles in society as well. Doing that, the organization addresses how men in our culture are trained to be emotionally repressed and in denial, which creates a lot of confusion and problems. Getting in touch with emotions can bring great insight, healing, and clarity for men. That's what it did for me.

Joining MKP also connected me to a nationwide support

structure of likeminded men. There's a level of trust before I even meet them. As we talk, we can quickly establish a relationship.

I also developed support structures in other parts of my life, focusing on things such as business, meditation, emotional intelligence, and Qigong. Those structures all had a weekly meeting on the same day and at the same time. Each meeting deepened connections and offered clarity of purpose. If I had problems, I caught them much quicker that way. It's an incredibly productive way to operate.

DAVID LANG

While I was still making sense of the insights from the retreat, I got an email out of the blue from David Lang.

I knew David through the ManKind Project. He lived across the country in San Diego, CA. He had heard about my issues through the grapevine and decided to reach out.

He said he had been in these woods before. He had been through stage 4 cancer and returned to health using integrated practices. After a complete recovery, he is now a triathlete and president of the National Triathlete Association.

He was just reaching out to see if I needed help. I emailed back and said, "Yes!"

We started talking. He shared sophisticated and brilliant insights.

One of his strategies was to get a "medical concierge." The medical concierge was a physician he had hired to be the quarterback for his cancer recovery team. The medical concierge could talk to his cardiologist, oncologists, naturopath, and whoever else he was working with. The concierge would then summarize it for David and say, "Here's what everyone is recommending. Here's what it means for you. Here are the side effects. Here's what I recommend." David would then choose his treatment path. It was a high-level way to deal with a serious illness.

I was inspired by his approach, but I decided to play that concierge role myself.

As medical concierge, I would be the general manager of my own healthcare team. I would decide who I wanted on the team. I would pick complementary members who would bring different insights and particular skills. Then I would coordinate them so everyone's on the same page. As the general manager, I would be the one making the decisions. Rather than a passive receiver of healthcare, I would be the one actually initiating and managing the process.

I laid out my game plan to Dr. Jung. He could have resisted my new approach, but instead he was openminded and curious. He said, "Not everyone does this. Let me know how it goes."

I also wanted to keep my allergist at Mayo in the loop, but I was afraid of being judged by him. I thought he would probably think this was quackery. I expected resistance. I didn't want to open it up to conversation and have him talk me out of it. I had gotten all the information I could from him, so I wasn't going to look to him for approval. So I just called and left a message with his assistant, a nurse who can be called any time. I informed her, "Here's what I'm going to do. I'll keep you posted." I didn't get resistance from her. I don't think I had a full discussion about my intentions with my allergist until after I had executed the plan.

I'm used to building expert teams in businesses and non-profits. I built my health recovery medicine team in the same way.

Obviously, the first person on my team was David Lang. I then brought on Dr. Jung and my allergist.

The next step would be to find a naturopathic doctor. David Lang is on the board at Bastyr University in Seattle, one of the few accredited naturopathic schools in the country. He introduced me to a faculty and board member there, Dr. Jane Guiltinan.

Dr. Guiltinan

I had a 30-minute phone consultation with Dr. Guiltinan. She was willing and helpful. We discussed my situation and she made some suggestions. She prescribed some herbal medicines to get me started.

Our second and last call was only ten minutes long. It was centered on supplies that I couldn't find locally. She said that Bastyr had a department from which I could order those supplements.

After both calls, I asked Dr. Guiltinan if I could compensate her, but she refused. It struck me how kind and service-oriented she was. She was extremely helpful and efficient.

Since Dr. Guiltinan was a full-time professor and didn't run a practice, she wasn't in a position to take me on as a patient. So she connected me with another board member, Dr. Carrie Louise Daenell, ND, who had a practice in Denver. Dr. Guiltinan and David Lang both had a high opinion of her.

Dr. Daenell

So I called and set up an appointment with Dr. Daenell. Afterwards, her office emailed a welcome letter and intake forms.

In that formulaic welcome letter, she congratulated me on my "decision to pursue a higher level of wellness." She set intentions to "provide personalized, compassionate wellness-consulting care." She would be my "resource for the 'best of the best' that natural medicine has to offer." She aimed "to stay on the cutting edge of the natural health field" and would "provide nutritional supplements of exceptional quality and bioavailability."

The intake forms were no less thorough than the one I had filled out at Mayo. Here's how those forms were described in that welcome letter:

They are extensive, as we have a healthy respect for the "whole person" in our practice. A full medical and symptom history is the beginning of this very individualized process. Please set aside ample time to fill out these forms and bring the completed copy with you to your initial appointment. Please bring any copies of lab work that you happen to have and please bring in all prescription and over the counter medications you are currently taking, along with any nutritional supplements.

I fastidiously filled out all the forms and provided all the information and documents requested in preparation for our appointment.

That appointment was a two-hour initial consultation by phone. In fact, our entire relationship would be over the phone.

That initial call was exploratory on both our parts. At the end, she might say, "I can't help you." I might say, "She's not for

26

me." It was understood that we were both kicking the tires.

She had looked through my medical records, so she knew about my asthma as a kid, how it had evolved as an adult and, of course, my respiratory breakdown of Christmas 2012.

After hearing what I had to say, she surprised me. She said, "After what you've told me, we can help you get better." No one else was telling me that. But she was clear: "You can get better. Not only can you get better, but you could even cure your asthma." No one had ever told me that. I didn't know whether to believe her. But her confidence impressed me, so I said, "Let's do this."

Dr. Daenell then added the caveat, "We can do things that will improve your situation. But you'll need to be committed. This could take between one and three years. But I've got a plan."

I was committed and highly motivated. It helped to have life or death on the line.

We had one-hour appointments via phone once every three months. During our appointments, we'd review how I was doing and go through a checklist. We'd look at whatever stage we were in and what was next.

We worked with the understanding that I would contact my local doctor about any pressing medical issue. She wasn't trying to subvert the system, but instead would supplement it.

There was nothing too oddball about working with her. Nothing seemed that strange, compared to conventional medicine. It was just the way she thought about my situation that was different. Unlike Jade...

Jade Nguyen

David highly recommended acupuncture, so I started making calls to find out what was available locally. A good friend whom I trust referred me to Jade Ngoc Nguyen.

Jade is a Vietnamese woman who practices Chinese medicine. She is a specialist who is trained in this — not just someone who has taken on acupuncture on the side.[8] She spent four years in Minneapolis at a school of Chinese medicine. She's confident and committed to the craft.

Jade's practice is located in a humble family-owned building. It has two treatment rooms and a little waiting area. There's a countertop reception desk that she runs herself. In the back half of the building, her mom runs a Vietnamese food store that also stocks herbal remedies.

Jade's English is good, but she has enough of an accent that I have to listen hard to understand her. What she's told me about Chinese medicine has been fascinating.

Jade does her entire diagnosis by holding my wrist, feeling my pulse, and looking at my eyes and tongue. That apparently tells her what she needs to know.

The first time she did that, I thought, "That was it? What could that have possibly shown?" She assured me that there were 22 different things she could identify that way. Even though it was a bit strange, I liked and trusted her right away. She was in.

---

[8] She is unlike many of the chiropractors in our area, who seem to have added acupuncture to have one more service to sell to their clients.

The Protocol

This was a strange new world, but I liked it because it was an adventure. It was fun. The people I encountered in it were dedicated and sincere.

I think it is important to note: I don't trust everyone. I trust only those people who are credible, committed, and have integrity.

There were a lot of well-meaning people in my life who told me to eat this or try that. They each recommended their pet solution. There were a lot of herbal remedies suggested. A juice sold through multilevel marketing was supposed to cure all problems. One of the stranger suggestions was eating the oats that are given to horses. There was no science or logical argument behind that one. It was just some urban legend.

But those well-meaning people weren't on the team, so I didn't pay much attention to them. I tuned them out so quickly that I don't remember many of their suggestions. I trusted my team and dismissed recommendations that weren't based on expertise.

I took the experts at their word. They gave me a brief explanation, but I just needed to know what they recommended. If they said a supplement or technique was good, I took their word on that. I went to trusted sources. Then I followed what the trusted sources recommended.

As I worked with my team, I assembled a list of expert recommendations, many of which felt counterintuitive.

I realized quickly that I was trying to do so many things at once that I had a hard time keeping them all straight. I had to establish a routine. I needed a cohesive system. So I developed an eight-point plan using the acronym: **B-R-A-I-N-N-S-S**:[9]

B - *Breathing*
R - *Running (and cardio)*
A - *Acupuncture*
I - *Ingestion*
N - *Nasal Lavage*
N - *Nebulize*
S - *Supplements*
S - *Sleep*

This gave me a checklist to use everyday.[10]

As I worked through these steps, I was still hyper-aware of not getting sick, which would be the beginning of another downward cycle. I washed my hands all the time. I avoided crowds. If I got a sniffle, a wheeze, or more phlegm in my lungs, I was quick to shut things down by staying home all weekend and sleeping in. I wasn't going to push it. I had no tolerance when it came to getting sick.

I would measure my progress with this B-R-A-I-N-N-S-S protocol in a few different ways:

· I would use a peak flow meter every morning to track my ability to push air out of my lungs. It was good for tracking progress and slippage.
· I would mark off each item on my daily checklist as I completed them.

---

[9] Much later, my editor would mock this acronym, saying "brains" pronounced this way (with two Ns and two Ss) sounded like a zombie.

[10] See: Appendix I: My Actual Daily Checklist

- When I got strong enough to exercise again, I would test myself every two weeks with a 10K run. My performance would tell me where I was. If I got faster, that would be exciting since it would mean I was getting healthier.

Both the ManKind Project and my Zen training encouraged setting clear intentions. Meditating, after all, is an attempt to gain clarity.

I set an intention, with the naturopath's support, for *complete respiratory restoration.* This is what I wanted, and I was willing to do whatever it takes.

At a time when my lungs were bad, after a lifetime of suffering from asthma, that was a compelling target. I didn't know if it was possible. The doctors had said the damage was probably permanent. But I understood how important it was to set intentions, so I decided to be ambitious and see what would unfold.[11]

I got everybody on my medical and personal support team on the same page for this target.

---

[11] It's worth noting that I wasn't attached to an outcome. I was just dedicated to going after that goal.

6

The Eight-Point Protocol

B is for Breathing

One of the things Dr. Daenell suggested I do was a technique called Buteyko breathing.

Dr. Jung had never heard of it. I had had health issues my entire life and had never seen it mentioned, even though it would be right up the alley of someone with asthma.

As I learned, this technique was developed by a Russian doctor, Konstantin Pavlovich Buteyko. It was simple: 1) Breathe out more than you breathe in. 2) Keep your mouth closed and always breathe through your nose.

Buteyko's theory is that asthmatics unconsciously breathe in more than they breathe out, so there's less carbon dioxide and more oxygen at the cellular level. There isn't enough carbon dioxide to make an efficient exchange with oxygen, so breathing out more than you breathe in improves that exchange and the oxygenation of your blood.

On one hand, that made sense to me. As an asthmatic, I always look for more air. On the other hand, I wondered why breathing out more than I breathed in would make any difference. But I didn't see any potential downside or harm that could come of it, so I decided to do it.

The breathing was easy to integrate with my meditation practice. It was the same except I breathed in for two counts, and out for three counts.

It was harder to breathe this way while exercising. Dr. Daenell told me to keep my mouth closed and to breathe out more than I breathe in. That was a challenge. If I ran hard enough, I wanted to open my mouth to breathe. Also, my nose got stuffed up when I exercised. So I wasn't able to breathe through my nose for much beyond a fast walk. I would end up gasping for air. But I trusted Dr. Daenell because she had used this technique with a high-level female triathlete to recover from a complete respiratory breakdown. So I persisted.

R is for Running (and cardio)

My goal was to do 30 minutes of cardio every day. For someone recovering, cardio seems to be key.

I stumbled onto this recommendation online from the Cleveland Clinic.

The Cleveland Clinic, whose heart program has ranked as the best in the nation for 20 years, is a big believer in cardio. Before they'll do heart surgery, overweight or out-of-shape patients must lose weight and meet a minimum cardio requirement. The clinic's success rates are fantastic since they eliminate a major cause of unsuccessful surgeries: patients who aren't physically prepared for the stress.

It could be 10 minutes at three different times. It didn't have to be done all at once.

A is For Acupuncture

I received acupuncture every week.

I had heard about this treatment for years but had never tried it. Without fearing death, I wouldn't have even considered it. It seemed way off the beaten path — It was a little too "woo woo" for me.

But I was the same way with massage. For years, I had heard, "Massages are great. You should get one." But I thought, *I have to leave my house, go to some strange place, and take my clothes off. Not for me.* Then, one year, Kay had a masseuse come to our house for my birthday. It was exquisite. Once I had that first massage, I got through my insecurities and the weirdness. After that, I wanted one every week.

Despite my resistance, I trusted acupuncture because it's ancient and has stood the test of time.

The theory behind Chinese medicine is that the body can heal itself. So if you're sick, it's because something is blocking your body's natural healing ability. So by removing those blockages, your body naturally heals itself.

At the time, it wasn't clear to me how needles remove those blocks. I still don't completely understand, but I wasn't too concerned. I didn't have to understand the mechanics. I figured I could afford to invest 30 minutes per week in a procedure that *might* work and wouldn't hurt me.

With acupuncture, Jade put needles in my forehead, chest, arms, stomach, legs, and feet. Then I would lie there for 20-30 minutes. Sometimes I would meditate during that time. Other times I would just nap. Then she would come back in and take out the needles, and I would go on my way.

Most of the time, the needles didn't hurt much. But one time, they ached. Jade said, "That's good. That's where you're blocked." So after that, when they hurt on occasion, I figured, "Okay, I guess that's good. This is where I'm blocked. I really need this one."

Every other time, she ended the session by burning a root called macta. She put the smoke near my skin and moved it around. It smelled somewhat like a cigar, and I could feel its heat.

I is for Ingestion

With ingestion, my goal was to become more conscious of what I put into my body. The plan was to maximize my body's ability to heal itself through food.

My ingestion approach came from an amalgamation of sources. The seed was planted by a book my late brother, David, had recommended. When Jade made recommendations, it was clear she was pointing toward the same approach. I also incorporated some conventional practices that are widely known and accepted.

Whereas most people despise diets, I was happy and excited. Of all the unknowns, I looked at what I was eating and thought, I can control that.

Water

Water is core. I drank 64 ounces of water a day. The first thing I did in the morning was drink a large glass of water. Then I drank another big glass before I leaving home. I took a 24-ounce plastic water bottle to work and drank that during the day. At night, I drank two more big glasses.

Drinking that much water allows the body to function well. I don't think that's a crazy insight. It's universally agreed upon. But what I didn't know at the time is that drinking lots of water can help thin the mucus in lungs, which allows the body to expel it more easily. I benefitted from this without even knowing it.

"Hot" Foods

Jade, although she was an acupuncturist, was helpful in cleaning up my diet.

Jade's view was that the American diet is perfect for blocking energy and impeding healing. Cheeseburgers, fried foods, and sugary beverages all create inflammation that accelerates the development of most ailments, including diabetes, heart disease, and cancer.

In her capacity as a Chinese medical practitioner, Jade's diagnosis was that my gut was "too hot." The "gut" is the power source for the immune system, and its effects radiate throughout the body. So if the digestive system runs too hot, it dries out the body and causes excess mucus formation in lungs. So "heat" creates mucus.

She told me to cut out beef, chicken, dairy, spicy food, and sweets. In her world, those are "hot" foods. So what does that leave? Surprisingly, I could eat pork. Pork is considered a "cool" meat. Fish, fruits, and vegetables are also fine.

So I had a much more plant-based diet. The only proteins I ate much of were fish and eggs.

She even prescribed boiling artichokes and then drinking the water as a coolant for my stomach. That was odd, but I was up for the adventure. I thought, *Artichoke water: How bad could it taste?* It turns out that it was pretty bad, but I drank it anyway.

I restricted my diet more and more. I cut out caffeine and sugar. I severely reduced my consumption of alcohol, fried foods, and salt.

The Anticancer Diet

The most influential book I've read on ingestion was *Anticancer: A New Way of Life* by David Servan-Schreiber. My late brother, David, had recommended it years earlier.

It's a well-written book by a neuroscientist who had a malignant brain tumor. Doctors removed the tumor, and he was considered cured. But because he didn't change his old lifestyle, the tumor came back. That's when he got serious and realized he had to do something drastic. It was the same kind of situation I found myself in.

Servan-Schreiber looked at cancer rates in Asia, India, and the Mediterranean, which were a tenth of what the U.S. had. His research led him to look at the diets of people in those regions.

Servan-Schreiber also talked about experiments in which rats were injected with cancer cells. Then, when bulging with tumors, they were injected daily with extracts of cruciferous vegetables like broccoli. The tumors shrank. Weirdness aside, the data pointed to a relationship between healing and a diet heavy in plant-based foods.

The most useful part of the book, for me, was that it ranked vegetables and fruits by their anticancer qualities. For example, broccoli and blueberries are both nutritional home runs. I wanted to focus on the foods that had the biggest impact, and his charts made it easy for me to do that.

Fruits and Vegetables

I ate at least five servings of fruits and vegetables a day, just as the USDA recommends.

Not only that, I ate fruits and vegetables particularly high in antioxidants: blueberries, strawberries, and cruciferous vegetables, e.g., broccoli, cauliflower, Brussels sprouts.

Because I'm not much into food preparation and because fresh produce spoils fast, I had to figure out a way to systematize it. My solution was buying frozen and dried fruits and vegetables.

At my office, I would eat a handful of prunes and dried apricots. They keep well and are tasty. So I easily got two out of five servings right there.

I would also microwave a large bag of frozen broccoli and split it up into four smaller containers. That was my salad base. Every day, I took a container, threw in a little spinach, a couple of cherry tomatoes, some chopped onions, and whatever else was around. Then I put a little salad dressing on it and closed it up. That was lunch.

Between those snacks and lunch, I had my five servings of fruits and vegetables taken care of.

Smoothies

I bought a Blendtec blender and made a lot of green smoothies with high-impact fruits and vegetables. They were delicious and easy to make.

I blended frozen blueberries, strawberries, pineapple, spinach, kale, whey protein powder, hemp seeds, chia seeds, and coconut milk. I also added water to make the smoothie easier to blend.

Each batch yielded about three servings. That was enough for Kay and my breakfast and my snack in the afternoon.

Bread

hile recovering, I cut out bread from my diet to reduce phlegm. I also avoided all standard grains, like wheat and rice.

However, during that time, I never stopped craving sandwiches and toast. The urge was strong.

N is for Nasal Lavage

I did nasal lavage every morning and every evening.

Nasal lavage, in layman's terms, is shooting saltwater up your nose. It clears out your sinuses. It clears out mucus as well as pollen and other allergens. Then the salt shrinks the swollen membranes that cause stuffiness.

The allergist at Mayo had actually recommended nasal lavage five years earlier, before all my latest health issues arose. But I never tried it because it sounded uncomfortable and weird. Then after I got sick, Dr. Daenell recommended it. So, with my health at stake, I made the plunge.

I went to a local drugstore and bought the device[12] for only $5. It's a plastic bottle with a nozzle. You unscrew the top and pour in a salt packet. Then you fill the water up to a certain level, put the nozzle on and shake it to create a saltwater solution. You then place the nozzle in one nostril and squeeze the bottle. The saltwater shoots up into your sinus and then comes out the other nostril. You repeat the same process with the other nostril.

Once the container is filled, it's all set for a week. It takes only 30 seconds to flush out the sinuses. The device required little maintenance. At the end of the week, I cleaned it out and set it up for the next seven days.

N is for Nebulize

Nebulizing is another technique that came from Dr. Daenell. Again, no one talked about this but her. I don't know how else I would've found out about it.

Nebulizing comes in many forms. In my case, nebulizing meant taking glutathione powder, mixing it with distilled water, and putting that into a device that turns the liquid into a mist. You then inhale the mist through one end of the tube and exhale out the other.

Glutathione is a favorite antioxidant of the naturopathic world for respiratory repair. I was already taking glutathione capsules as part of my supplements (see next section). But this procedure would be even more powerful since it would directly

---

[12] Neti pots function differently but serve the same purpose. I used the NeilMed Sinus Rinse, but any device that rinses out the nasal passages is fine.

apply the antioxidant to my damaged lungs.

Even though I trusted my team, this was scary. If the device wasn't kept sterile, I could breathe in an irritant. In my fragile condition, I could kill myself if I inhaled infectious agents into my damaged lungs.

I was afraid, but I did it anyway.

The first step was finding glutathione powder. The problem is that you can't go to just any pharmacy and buy it. It had to be obtained from a sterile compounding pharmacy, and there aren't too many of them in the country. Dr. Daenell recommended one in San Diego, but their license didn't allow them to sell to Iowa. So I had to look around. That step alone took a couple of months to figure out. Fortunately, I eventually found a pharmacy 90 minutes away that took my order.

Then I had to figure out how to run the machine. To make the device work, there was some assembly required. The first time I used the nebulizer, it started bubbling all over the place and made a mess. It was like putting too much soap in the dishwasher. I called the lab and told them how it hadn't gone well. They said, "You probably put too much water in there. Try it with less water and see how you do." They were right.

There was a lot of cleanup and preparation. I nebulized twice a day, and each session took about an hour: to put the device together, inhale the mist, break down the device, and sterilize it.

S is for Supplements

While I was depending on only conventional medicine, I took these seven supplements daily: Centrum Silver Multi-vitamin (for adults 50+), vitamin C, vitamin D, aspirin, Omega 3, EPA, and acidophilus (a probiotic).

The list of supplements the naturopaths wanted me to take in addition to these was extensive. Dr. Guiltinan recommended adding three supplements: NAC (N-Acetyl-L-Cysteine), Ivy Calm, and Herbal Respiratory Relief. Dr. Daenell approved of all of those and added nine more supplements: HistArrest, QuerceMax, Vital D, Lyprinol, Celleration, Q Right, BioMax, Detox Essentials, and IgG 2000 DF.

Dr. Daenell printed out a list with the recommended dosages. Since she had a system where she got high-quality ingredients from several sources, I bought much of my supplements through her.[13]

These herbal remedies assisted the natural healing of my body in different ways, but I couldn't say what each supplement did specifically for the healing process.

The majority of these supplements, like vitamins, were in capsule form. A few were powders that were mixed with water for drinking.

There were also supplements that I took on an as-needed basis. Jade recommended the Chinese herb *ding chuan wan* for two weeks to calm my asthma, clear heat, and reduce phlegm.

It's worth noting that these supplements didn't replace my current prescription medications. These were additional.

Since it was a big list, I learned to make up six days' worth of doses at one time and put them in little containers. I would then take the contents of the container at the appropriate time. Certain supplements I took in the morning, and others in the evening. Once sorted, it was a streamlined process. It took only two minutes, twice daily, to take them all with a big glass of

---

[13] To some, this may seem like a red flag because she could have had a profit incentive. But I trusted that Dr. Daenell had my best interests at heart.

water.[14]

I could see where my pill regimen might be incomprehensible for people who struggle to consistently take a daily multivitamin. But I was used to taking medications on a regular basis. With the corticosteroid inhaler, I had taken puffs every morning and evening for 30 years. Consuming medication on a daily basis was already a well-ingrained habit. I was just adding to my list of medications. It was the same routine, though I now had many more bottles of pills.

S is for Sleep

We're in a country that's famous for people who burn the midnight oil. However, sleep is fundamental to the immune system.

Sleep wasn't so much something I implemented in my protocol. It was something that my body demanded. I was

---

[14] You may be wondering, since I was my own medical concierge and not a master of chemistry, how I integrated all these supplements from multiple sources and still felt safe. I'll admit it — it could have been a mistake. It could have been dangerous in a way I didn't understand. Any complications, even an allergic reaction, would have been damaging. Everything I took was herbal ... but so is hemlock. I was clearly taking risks, yet I didn't put much effort into understanding these supplements. With Detox Essentials, for example, I didn't know what's in it or how it works. But I assured myself that I was working with knowledgeable professionals.

Before taking anything, I always looked up the ingredients in the supplements and consulted with Dr. Jung. I had him look at each one and say, "This is okay." So, I did some due diligence by checking each supplement with a traditional medical practitioner who's trained in chemistry and biology. That process probably wasn't very thorough, but it was all I asked for at the time.

so wiped out by my illness, my self-prescribed regimen, and my business that it was hard to stay awake. I slept 12 to 14 hours per day. In addition to the hours I slept at night, I also napped one to two hours in the afternoon. That much sleep was necessary for me just to feel okay and have a minimal amount of energy.

Before this experience, I ran a high-intensity, high-achievement lifestyle. I would get tired, but I would push through. Skimping on sleep was unsafe, but it didn't feel unsafe at the time. I did this because I had a sense that I wasn't enough and hadn't done enough. So something more always needed to happen. I would routinely go beyond what was safe or healthy for my body. For my whole life, I pushed myself and did more, even when I was tired. I would wear myself out and get sick. That was part of what got me into this situation.

So I just decided I wasn't going to fight my sleepiness. I would surrender to that fact and sleep when I needed to sleep.

Kay supported my sleep schedule. She said, "You sleep as much as you need to. You've just got to do it. You don't have a choice."

7

Running The Protocol

I started developing the protocol in June 2013. It's not like I got this out of a ready-made kit. I didn't open up a box and pull all the parts out. It took me about until August to have everything collected and codified.

Even though I now had my team and my protocol, it was still a long road back to Mayo for my one-year checkup.

I now had a solid plan for recovery, but I wasn't immune to despair. Three months into the protocol, I wrote the following journal entry:

> *Got a cold. The phlegm has turned from milky white to light green — that's the danger signal. Feeling anger, sadness, and fear. Fear of death. I don't want to die... yet.*

I went through a lot of doubt and personal struggle during this process. I didn't know if what I was doing would work. With no established route to follow, I was cutting my own path in this dark wilderness.

Instituting my protocol, my days shrunk. Following B-R-A-I-N-N-S-S swallowed up four hours every day, and that's not counting the 12–14 hours of sleep. I worked for three to four hours. My remaining waking hours were minimal.

I went to bed at 8 p.m. and woke up between 8 and 10 a.m. In the summer, I slept from dusk until after dawn.

I had no social life. Evenings were spent at home. It wasn't like I had to leave parties early. There *were* no parties. Getting well took priority over everything else.

Let's say I needed only 12 hours of sleep. This is what a typical day looked like:

> *8–8:30 a.m. — Wake up, eat breakfast, and get ready for the day*
> *8:30–10:30 a.m. — Morning protocol of nebulization, nasal lavage, taking supplements, and cardio*
> *10:30–11 a.m. — Drive to the office*
> *11 a.m.–2 p.m. — Work and eat lunch at my desk*
> *2–3 p.m. — Take a nap[15]*
> *3–4 p.m. — Work some more*
> *4:30–5 p.m. — Drive home*
> *5–7 p.m. — Evening protocols of more nebulizing, more nasal lavage, and more supplements*
> *7–8 p.m. — Eat dinner with Kay and watch a TV show together*
> *8 p.m. — Climb into bed*

My weekends were pretty similar, though I had more time to

---

[15] I had a couch put in my office so I could lie down whenever I needed to. Napping was the way I made it through the day and got enough energy to do the next task.

enjoy a leisurely breakfast. In the afternoons, Kay and I would go out and do something together.

Kay appreciated how I was focused and serious about recovering, but it was hard on our relationship because I had less time to spend with her. At the same time I was doing my protocol, her mother was dying. This period was extremely hard on Kay. She was worried about both her mom and me, but she didn't have a lot of support. I tried to be as supportive as I could be given the circumstance.

After instituting the protocol, it became clear that business as usual wouldn't cut it anymore. Adopting the protocol completely restructured my life. It made my waking hours dearer than ever.

I was left with about four hours per day to operate as president of my investing firm. In addition to my leadership role, I was — alongside my partner Corey — one of the primary client contacts, the primary research analyst, and a portfolio manager. My responsibilities were enough to fill a 40-hour workweek, but I now had to accomplish them in 20 or fewer hours.

Tim Ferriss, a productivity expert, put forth a thought experiment in his book *The 4-Hour Workweek*: "If you had a heart attack and had to work two hours per day, what would you do?"

This hypothetical case helps us remember that "simplicity requires ruthlessness. If you had to stop 4 / 5 of time-consuming activities... what would you eliminate to keep the negative effect on income to a minimum?"

Although I didn't have a heart attack, this scenario wasn't hypothetical for me. There would be no more goofing around.

That time constraint taught me to focus and prioritize. I realized I might have only a few years left, and I had only a few hours in the day. Time was valuable, so I always had to focus on the single most important thing. That single thing had to be done immediately because if I didn't, I would have wasted my one opportunity. There wouldn't be any energy or time to do it later.

Certain things never made my top priority, so they were cut. If it wasn't absolutely essential to business, it was gone.

I became acutely aware of just how much fluff I carry around in the workday. Many people, including me, crave this illusion of busyness. It shows our own importance when we have so much more that needs to be done. But it's amazing how much of that excess falls away the second you don't have time for it.

I was amazed at how much I could get done in one or two hours. Having a metaphorical gun to my head helped me learn to focus. That was a learning experience I wouldn't have had otherwise.

I like the word "ruthlessness" in describing this period. I had neither the time nor energy for messing around. No half measures would do.

Before this experience, there was a piece of me that desperately wanted to fit in, be liked, and wanted by others. I hadn't accepted myself. I had given myself up so I could fit in.

But radical self-acceptance was required now. I wouldn't be able to rely on the approval of others and still be able to do what needed to be done. The ruthlessness required to do this protocol might leave others feeling cut off or disconnected. I had to accept that.

In making myself the priority, I could no longer be a people pleaser. In fact, I was asking other people to make *me* the main priority. Well, I wasn't asking. I was informing people that I —

really, my health — was going to be the top priority.

It's hard to know what others thought of me at that time. If they were unhappy, they kept it to themselves. But I'm sure my team co-workers wanted more work from me than I was giving. I'm sure Kay wanted more of me than merely the last hour at the end of the day. I declined nearly every social engagement. Someone was getting less than they wanted from me at every step.

Even though I knew ruthlessness was the right thing for me to do at that time, it was still difficult. I wanted to connect, to be wanted. Part of me would have rather died than not be a part of what's happening. However, wanting to be a part of everything contributed to my near-fatal illness. I pushed myself too far, got run down, and almost died.

This ordeal was a wake-up call. It was the death of Mr. Nice Guy.

As months passed on this demanding schedule, I kept grinding through day by day, working hard to stay on track and not get derailed. This was the make-or-break point. A lot of people make positive changes (like diets), start feeling healthier, and then fall off the wagon.

Plenty of times, I wanted to quit my protocol. I wanted to stay at work to finish a task or stay up later to spend time with Kay.

There were definitely things I missed out on.

Kay and I used to love going up on top of our hill, with wine and cheese, to watch the sunset. This simple act of enjoying each other's company at the end of the day was squeezed out. It's not like I was missing a trip to the Super Bowl. I couldn't even go outside to enjoy the sunset.

For more than a decade, I had been part of a weekly ManKind Project group. But I had to stop attending meetings because they were held at night, and I simply couldn't stay up that late.

One thing I did not cut out was my weekly meditation group. I scheduled my day around being awake for the evening session. I carefully planned my energy and took a longer nap to make sure I could be there at 7:30 p.m.

That one session a week was all I could manage anymore. Before I got sick, my morning routine included 30 minutes of meditation, followed by Qigong. That was out. Even though I still highly valued meditation, there was no time for staring at a flame when I barely had time to see my wife.

We only had an hour to be together each day. We couldn't engage with the mundane day-in, day-out details of each other's lives. During my protocol, I remember listening to her talk. It took a lot less energy to do that. But she is a private person who internalizes things rather than sharing them, even with me.

Right before my health issues became severe, my marriage was full of beauty. Then, as the sickness moved in and her mother got ill, we went through a two-year valley of darkness.

It was an intense, stressful period. Our relationship was up and down for a long time.

That autumn, Kay's mother fell and broke her hip. After she got out of the hospital, she was moved into a nursing home. I would have liked to have gone there with Kay, but I couldn't. For me, nursing homes were Disease Central. As much as I wanted to be supportive, being around potentially sick people was a high-risk thing to do, so I stayed home.

I was so deep in my own struggle that even though I cared about Kay, she was demoted. I wasn't as available for her. I was available only for myself. There were times I could tell she resented it. There was a tension that we didn't discuss.

We each had our things we had to do. We supported each other as best we could, but we were largely on our own. I hardly saw her. She hardly saw me.

With Kay in her deep grief, I understood that following the protocol was up to me. I wasn't going to be able to rely on her for support. We didn't discuss this, but it became clear to me as we went along.

In my diminished state, I had to be self-reliant. I filled up the salt water for the nasal lavage. I counted out the pills. I cleaned out the nebulizer after each usage. I handled everything on my protocol.

I wasn't thinking any more than one step ahead. I narrowed my vision to my next action.

Even with those frustrations, even when things sucked, I went on anyway. There was no way out of the woods except to keep walking.

Previously, I resisted doing things that are new, odd, or just out of my normal experience. Now here I was with this unconventional protocol. Much of it no one had ever heard of. I did it despite what anyone else thought. I didn't care if it was weird. I didn't care anymore.

For example, I'm not sure I would have taken esoteric Chinese herbs for a cold before this experience. But this wasn't the normal course of events. Now a cold could quickly become an emergency. The risk-reward balance had shifted. A cold was now a much bigger risk, so I was willing to take chances with supplements.

Parts of me died: My indecisiveness. The part that knew what to do but didn't do it. The part that was put off by the nasal lavage pump looking weird. The part that let little things stand in his way.

Extreme circumstances forced the change I may have wanted to make but didn't have the motivation or strength to make otherwise.

I had known about nasal lavage five years before I tried it. I had read *The Anticancer Diet* the year before and had done a little with it, but I hadn't committed. I should've been eating five servings of fruits and vegetables a day. I should've been drinking that much water anyway. I should've been eating well regardless of my health.

But I wouldn't have changed my diet without death as a motivator. Being near death prompted me to clean up my diet, get proper sleep, and exercise. It would have been nice if it didn't require such high stakes and urgency to change. But it was necessary for me.

Luckily, the stakes were high enough that I blew through things that normally would have impeded me. I didn't have the time to be picky. The sense of urgency overwhelmed any resistance.

To remain on track, I hung up my daily checklist in my bathroom, kitchen, and office to make sure I was checking items off every day.

My priority was clear and never wavered. Every day I focused on the task in front of me.

I executed it at a high level, but I don't want to claim I was 100% perfect every day. Expecting that level of perfection can be intimidating. Instead, I did my best. I occasionally forgot to take certain supplements, but as I established a better pattern, it didn't happen often. If I was going to miss anything, it was cardio. I would miss it if I didn't have enough time in the morning to squeeze it in.

Sometimes things fell through, but overall I accomplished most things most days.

8

Measuring my Progress

It was a long, slow, gradual — but upward — journey through those eight months between when I implemented the protocol and my one-year checkup at Mayo.

I tested myself daily with a simple breath flow meter that Mayo had given me. I breathed in as much as I could and blew into the nozzle as hard as I could.[16] As you blow, your breath lifts raises a ball, much like the carnival game where you try to ring the bell. The higher the ball goes, the better your breath flow is. If I couldn't get the ball above the 500 mark, it meant my lungs weren't operating well enough. At the beginning of my protocol, I was well below 500.

Cardio was another indicator. I would track my capabilities with how long and how much I could exercise.

I was starting with nothing. At the lowest point of my health, I couldn't even walk down the stairs. On a scale of 1 to 100, my energy level was at about 7 when I started the protocol. I was so weak that I felt like an 85-year-old man.

---

[16] An unintentional benefit of using the flow meter was that it helped expel mucus from the lungs. Big breaths in and out act as huffing, which sometimes shakes mucus loose.

Obviously, I couldn't go straight from shuffling to jogging. So I started by walking.

The first time on the treadmill, my heart was racing after walking slowly for ten minutes. That's how far I had fallen. Ten minutes was my max.

I kept at it, though. After ten minutes of walking, I would rest. Then I would do another ten.

On one hand, I was expending energy. Exerting energy and saving up energy seemed like opposing forces. If I could barely get out of bed after 14 hours, how could I be expected to exercise?

But, on the other hand, cardio also created a vibrancy. To be active — feeling myself move, feeling the warmth generated from exercise, and even sweating — felt important.

Using an elliptical machine was the next step. It wasn't quite as strenuous as running, but it was more strenuous than walking. It was a good intermediary activity. I could more easily maintain proper breathing with that.

I then ventured outside. I could walk the 3-mile forest covered trip around a local lake name Bacon Creek in about 45 minutes.

I decided I was now ready to try running it.

I could easily do the Buteyko breathing while meditating and walking, but not while running. At some point while running, I would be forced to start breathing through my mouth. It wasn't optimal, but I did as much as I could. I would start out breathing the correct way, and then when I reached my limit, I would switch to mouth breathing so that I wouldn't have to stop.

Breathing through my nose while running was inhibited by my stuffiness. Therefore any improvement in clearing up my sinuses would translate into huge improvements with my Buteyko breathing.

The effect of nasal lavage was immediate. The first time I did it, it was like parting the Red Sea. After I did it, I immediately breathed better. It was a clear cause and effect. I was amazed how much of my stuffiness went away. I had been living with that stuffiness for 30 years without realizing I could've done something about it. Since my membranes had been in a state of constant irritation, I hadn't even been aware of how stuffed up I was until I started using the device. Over the weeks that followed, my membranes shrank more and more, and my passageways opened. Gradually, the inflammation in my sinuses was reduced.

By opening up my nasal passageways, I could run longer without getting to that gasping point. If I didn't do my nasal lavage before running, I couldn't go very far before I had to gasp for air.

As I figured out nebulizing, I still had a lot of fear that potentially inhaling an infection might create a setback in my health. Luckily, the procedure started to help right away. Nebulizing coagulated my phlegm, which made it easier to cough up. Gradually, my lungs got clearer and clearer. Soon there was less phlegm to expel. Also, after a nebulizing session, I usually felt really calm. There's a meditative quality to inhaling the mist.

I always timed my runs around Bacon Creek. After I started nebulizing, I dropped a couple of minutes right away. Whatever breaths I was taking, the oxygen exchange was more efficient, and I was able to run faster.

When I exercised, I could do more. My lungs were functioning at a higher level.

By changing my diet, I lost 15 pounds without even thinking about it. I got lighter and healthier. By staying with my new diet and adding whole foods, I felt a noticeable difference. I soon realized that the foods I used to put in my body were responsible for much of my problem. There was a relationship between certain foods and how much mucus I produce, but I had never made the connection between the two. The minute I changed, I became aware of how my diet could reduce or increase the amount of mucus in my lungs.

After staying on the diet for a while, I tried to add back bread. Unfortunately, bread creates phlegm for me, and it was clear that I was not doing my health any favors by eating it. I love bread, but I had to do what worked for me. And bread didn't work. When I tried reintroducing a number of other foods I removed, the result was also more mucus. I now realize that I had worked against myself for 30 years by eating hamburgers and dairy products. I had been creating a lot of my mucus through the foods I was eating, yet I had no awareness of it.

Dr. Daenell sent me a "leaky gut" test through the mail. The process was simple enough. I gave a urine sample, drank water with certain sickeningly sweet sugars mixed in, and then gave a second urine sample. Comparing the before and after results showed how well I processed those sugars and how efficient my digestive system was. I got a C– on that initial test. C– is only a little below baseline, but it still wasn't great. There was still work to do.

Initially, the supplements from Dr. Daenell specifically addressed respiratory repair. After the test, she shifted the focus to gut repair. She put me on another program of supplements, varying the mixture a bit. Like Jade, Dr. Daenell believed the gut to be the center of the immune system, and a healthy gut allows the body to heal itself.

As for acupuncture, I don't know if it had an effect at all. Perhaps I'm not sensitive enough to know. I couldn't really see the results, but I didn't see any harm, either.

I don't remember huge breakthrough days. I just kept at it, and my energy and running speed gradually improved. Of course, there were occasional setbacks, but overall, my performance trended up.

Energy was essential in my cardio. It takes energy to exercise. On days when I felt exhausted, I wouldn't exercise and would sleep instead. Some days I couldn't wait to exercise. It felt great. Some days I felt tired, and it was a push. Other days, I felt so tired that I couldn't even force myself. I had to surrender to my fatigue and sleep, whereas before I used to push through. During my recovery, I had to honor my body and whatever it was asking for.

Over time, I felt more and more energetic after exercising. I was getting more energy over time.

After eight months of following the protocol, my energy was at about 70%. I was consistently blowing over 500 on the breath flow meter. But it would still vary. When I caught a cold, for example, the number would drop below 500.

I had to stay with the Buteyko breathing technique for a long time to see an effect, but it worked for me. Slowly, I became less wheezy, my lungs began to clear, and there was less and less mucus.

The improvement in my breathing from the Buteyko technique seemed even more profound in the light of cardio. I was running those three miles around Bacon Creek in about ten-minute miles. I could run for two miles before I had to breathe through my mouth.

I hadn't broken through yet, but I could feel this was all building toward something.

9

Returning to Mayo

The moment had arrived. April 2014 marked a year since the original diagnosis. It was time to return to Mayo for my one-year checkup.

Twelve months earlier, Kay had driven the five hours to take me to Mayo. I slept in the passenger seat almost the entire way. When we got there, I was so tired that I had no qualms about sleeping on the floor of the busy lobby while waiting to get tested. I remember looking at Kay. She looked haggard and exhausted. My ordeal had taken a toll on her as well. I was in a slightly better mood than her because I enjoyed the attention.

Returning to Mayo, one year later, I was the one who drove. We stayed at a nice hotel, and I saw it as a weekend getaway with my wife.

Kay was nervous, but nothing like before. I felt good, but I was still nervous.

I didn't know how these tests would go, but I was confident they'd be better.[17] I just didn't know how much better. I knew

---

[17] The month prior, I had just had a full physical with Dr. Jung. All of the tests were in the normal range except cholesterol, which had elevated from 186 to 197. So no spectacular news there.

with these protocols that I was healthier. So, regardless of what the test said, I was going to keep doing them.

I didn't know how much of my lung damage was permanent. Even feeling better, there could be things that I wouldn't be able to get over.

I knew the good, but I didn't know the bad.

There is the feeling at Mayo that you're in someone else's system. You check in at the desk. They tell you to wait. Then they send you to another room. Then they do a test. Then they send you back. Then they send you somewhere else. You are a subordinate. You end up surrendering to their system.

Mayo is made up of dedicated, skilled, and intelligent doctors who take great pride in what they do. So I hesitated to say that I disagreed with them. I wanted to be right, but my insecurity said, "What hubris I must have? Who am I to say they were wrong?"

Still, I felt excited by my mission. That mission overrode my insecurities and my fears of looking foolish or insulting them. I wanted to see the fruits of my labor.

First, they did a pulmonary function test. My score was the best it had been since 2011. Not only had I recovered, I was healthier than I was in 2012. They were pleased and delighted.

Then they took a CAT scan to see where the lung damage was. Whiteness on the scan corresponded to inflammation. They told me that the thicker the whiteness, the more likely the tissue was damaged. Previously, six areas had been milky-white.

The pulmonologist compared each of six images to the corresponding milky-white ones from the year before.

He said "hmm…" after each one. I could tell he was surprised — and more than a little puzzled.

Each time he looked at the current scan, there was nothing. Not a speck. It was as clear as the night sky.

When he finished, he looked at me and asked, "So, what have you been doing?"

It was a miracle.

There was nothing there. There was no inflammation. There was no damaged tissue.

When the CAT scan came back clear, I almost cried. I was so joyful. It was the best possible outcome. He was happy for me and completely surprised. Neither of us had expected this outcome.

My *optimistic* estimate was that recovery would take years, if it was going to happen at all. So, having it happen so quickly — in about eight months — was surprising.

I now saw my chance to show the experts what I had done. I pulled out a diary of everything I did, when I did it, who I met with, and the results I measured. The diary included calls to the naturopath, visits to the acupuncturist, the breathing technique, supplements, and so on. All of it was typed up in the diary.

The pulmonologist flipped through it and said, "Ahh. Acupuncture. Yeah, that can help. Naturopathy? No. That doesn't do anything."

I was still so happy. At least, I wanted to be happy. But there was a part of me that wanted to confront him and say, "Now wait a minute. This outcome is beyond anything you could've expected. Aren't you at least curious to know more about what I think worked?"

But I was so overwhelmed by the news that I didn't challenge him. There's a part of me that wishes I had said, "How do you explain what you saw? At least, be open."

I get it. He's coming from a world of thorough testing, measurement, history, and experience. In that world, you don't consider anything unless it has a comprehensive body of empirical evidence behind it. My approach was largely outside of that. I understood that. But I still wanted to say, "Well, this breathing technique is free. Why not, at least, try it before you rule it out?"

On the bright side, my protocol is now on file at Mayo. Even though I didn't fight him, I went fully on the record. I was completely transparent. Whether or not that medical establishment ever wants to accept my experience, I gave them the opportunity.

I felt complete.

I had withheld information when I decided to take this route initially. I evaded my allergist and left a note with his assistant. So it was cathartic to just know that all my documentation is on file there.

I didn't need them to sign off on it. I didn't need them to approve of it. I didn't need a gold star from the authority figures like I had always needed before. The doctor said naturopathy doesn't work. I didn't buy it — not even for a moment. His resistance in no way swayed me. It's on him if he doesn't want to see it, but I'm not going to hide it or pretend.

10

An Anticlimactic Celebration

I was validated that I had beaten death (at least temporarily — life is impermanent, after all).

I was joyful, but it was also an anticlimactic moment. We didn't have a party to celebrate. Kay's mom's passing the previous month was front and center. It weighed heavy on that moment.

But I did call David Lang and other allies from the ManKind Project. As I told the whole story, I felt joyful, heard, and supported. David was happy for me. He had taken a risk reaching out to me, an acquaintance at the time. He didn't know what was going to happen to me. I expressed my gratitude to him for starting me on this path. I couldn't have done it without him.

Another reason this was anticlimactic was that my recovery had all been so gradual. So it wasn't like one day I was dying and the next day I was okay. It was a long, slow, incremental climb to where I was now. The great news was just validation of how I already felt.

Nonetheless, I was excited to share the news with Dr. Daenell.

When I called Dr. Daenell, she was thrilled the tests had gone so well.

I told her about how the pulmonologist had said that naturopathy doesn't do anything. She said, "Yeah. They tend to feel that way."

She was not surprised by the resistance I received. She has dealt with the conventional medical world enough to be disappointed over and over by its practitioners' lack of openness to her naturopathic worldview.

I said, "But you're in the system now. That file is in there."

The next phase after Mayo was a follow-up leaky gut test with Dr. Daenell. Last time, my score was low (C-). Now, after having spent months following her gut repair program, it was time to retest to see if there was any improvement.

This time, I got an A. My gut had rebounded. My immune system was much stronger.

Two months later, Dr. Daenell and I met in person for the one and only time.

I was flying through Denver on my way home from a wedding in San Francisco. She was arriving there after a trip to Italy. We would have a moment of overlap to meet before I caught my connecting flight.

I was excited to see this person who was so important to me and whose disembodied voice I had spent hours with over the phone.

Then, her flight was delayed and mine started boarding. It didn't seem like we would be able to see each other.

Rushing over, she was able to get to my gate just before I boarded.

There she was — shorter than I expected, wearing a dark

brown leather jacket, looking worn out from traveling for hours, with tears in her eyes. This woman, standing in front of me, had helped me not die. She had hope for me when no one else did.

Before she said anything, I was overwhelmed with gratitude. I reached out and gave her a big hug. I told her how much I appreciated her. I was so effusive, open, and grateful that it surprised her.

After only two minutes together, the airport called final boarding. I gave her another big hug and wished her well.

As I walked down the platform to the plane, I felt a total sense of victory. "We did it. It worked. It actually worked!"

11

Epilogue: 18 Months Later

Since I received great news, it may seem like my struggle is over. But as filmmaker Orson Welles once said, "If you want a happy ending, that depends, of course, on where you stop your story."

My story isn't over.

I haven't completely shut this out. Bronchiectasis could always come back. I have to stay vigilant.

Remembering those low moments keeps me sharp. I never want to go back to where I was, with lungs full of mucus and gasping for every breath. That motivates me to stay with this healthy lifestyle. I never want to forget where I'll wind up if I don't.

It's not that I had bronchiectasis once, got over it, and never have to worry about getting it again. I'm still vulnerable. This condition will hang over my head for the rest of my life. I need to be careful and focused, day to day, on not getting sick.

The downward spiral is always possible.

I think there's such a thing as healthy paranoia. I have that.[18] I'm always concerned about my immune system. Now when I get run down, I am much quicker to get to bed, sleep, and recover. I no longer wait until the symptoms get worse, like I did in my younger years.

I still heed the original "Be careful" warning. I wash my hands often. If I'm in a crowded area or if people are touching stuff, I keep my hands to myself. I try to be smart about not contracting diseases.

I still wear a mask on airplanes. I'm usually the only one on the plane who does that. I see how people look at me. They must think, "Does he have a contagious disease? Is he going to infect me?"

I could be seen as weird, but that doesn't bother me anymore. The person I'm traveling with may say, "People are looking at us." I'll think, *Yeah, this is an odd thing to do. Oh well.* It may make my friend feel uncomfortable, but I'm completely at peace with that too.

I'm not going to risk death just to keep strangers or even friends from feeling uncomfortable.

I don't care about what other people think and whether they object. What I'm doing is right for me. I will protect my health whether they like it or not.

In healing myself, I saw my recovery as validation of this integrated path. I'm paying more attention to my health, my body, and my life.

I am inspired to maximize my body's ability to heal itself

---

[18] In my journal, I had actually written the phrase "had visitation/funeral without picking up something." Yes, I was relieved that I went to a wake and didn't become ill. That shows where my mind was.

through good nutrition, exercise, and a healthy lifestyle. I have recovered to the point where I am better than where I was when I started. But it's not about getting back to where I started. I'm going to see how far this new path can take me and how far I can go in improving my health.

Eighteen months after seeing Dr. Daenell at the Denver airport, I'm still following the protocol, though I'm not as rigorous as I once was.

I still do Buteyko breathing while meditating and exercising.

Meditation and Qigong are daily practices. I spend at least 30 minutes meditating and doing Qigong in the morning. If I have time on the weekends, I mediate an hour and do a half-hour of Qigong.

I still do 30 minutes of cardio every day. I am continuing to improve my running times.

Earlier this year, I decided to challenge myself to do a 10K[19] on the treadmill. My goal was to do it in an hour. But more importantly, I just wanted to go that far. Even if I had to walk, I wanted to go to the full 6.2 miles. Amazingly, I was able to run all the way through, doing Buteyko breathing, in 63 minutes. At a ten-minute-per-mile pace, that's the best I've run in the last decade.

As I recovered, Jade started ramping down the frequency of our acupuncture visits. She said I only needed to come back if and when I got sick.

I haven't done acupuncture for over six months because Jade phased it out as I recovered. She said to come as needed, and I haven't felt the need.

---

[19] 6.2 miles

My diet is more relaxed. I eat *forbidden foods* from time to time. In moderation, I have eaten pizza, sandwiches, and toast — and thoroughly enjoyed each one. But these moments are the exception rather than the rule. I eat bread far less than I once did.

I have an ongoing struggle with sweets in my diet. Part of me doesn't want to be disciplined. I want to eat cakes, pies, and cookies. So it helps that when I eat those sweet things, my body responds poorly and I don't feel as good.

I still drink huge amounts of water.

I eat an increasingly plant-based diet.

I'm getting better at eating fresh vegetables — not just dried and frozen ones. Kay and I have a CSA (Community Supported Agriculture) membership, so every week we get a bag of whatever is in season locally.

I still regularly consume foods high in antioxidants. Most days, I eat blueberries, strawberries, and cruciferous vegetables.

I still do the smoothies from time to time, but not consistently.

I still avoid Jade's "hot" foods of beef, chicken, and dairy. I don't eat much pork either, even though it's a "cool" meat. My protein is mostly from fish, eggs, and whey protein shakes.

I still do nasal lavage, but now only once per day instead of twice.

I haven't nebulized in a few months. That was phased out as well.

I figured I would have to nebulize forever because my situation was so bad. After a while, I got it down to where I needed to do it only once a day. Now I do it as needed (when mucus flares up), which isn't often.

I still take supplements every day, but it's a much shorter list (only 12 capsules daily).

Of all the things I lost, my energy took the longest to rebound. Dr. Daenell said it was a function of the immune system being so depleted. But I slowly got more energy.

I now need only eight hours of sleep to be recharged. I usually go to bed at 10 p.m. — just like I did before all of this started.[20]

I work a normal workday (8:30 a.m. to 5 p.m.) and leave feeling good at the end.

Afternoon naps during my workday are optional, but I still take them once in a while.

I feel less fatigued now, which means my immune system is healthier. I did not get sick for a whole year. The one time I got a cold, I bounced back quickly.

I still do the breath flow meter once in a while, but not every day. It's been in the 550–600 range for a long time. I've gotten it over 600 a few times. If it ever dropped below 500, that would sound an alarm, and I would monitor it more closely. But this hasn't happened.

Drying up the mucus took a long time. If I get any mucus at all, I now proactively address it. I clean up my diet, get more

---

[20] During my health struggle, my days had an immense clarity. I was a soldier with clear marching orders. I knew where to go, what to do, and when to do it. Since then, I've lightened up on my hyper level of focus. There is a little more horsing around. I'm not just knocking out the most important thing and then going home. Although I love my new life, I do miss that clarity. Everything is now freer, but with less direction.

During the worst of my health issues, the business didn't just maintain. It continued to grow and improve. After the dust settled, it was a record year. My office team had helped me carry the ball. I maximized my limited time with my increased focus, but I couldn't have done it without them.

sleep, and tighten up the protocol.

I used to have phlegm all the time. I didn't think twice about that for 30 years. Just like the stuffiness, I became blind to the phlegm. It felt like a normal part of everyday life. Now it's gone.

I'm less wheezy than I used to be. My lungs and nose are clear.

I feel better and my body feels younger than before I got sick.

In slowly clawing my way back, as a byproduct, I have nearly eliminated my asthma, a "permanent condition" I've had my entire life. I wanted to not die, and somehow I got rid of something I had even when I was "healthy."

This experience has changed me, and not just physically. It has affected the rest of my life. I feel lighter, less attached, and more joyful.

Before my illness, I thought I was at peace with my mortality. But without this illness, I don't think I would have found out how much further I had to go. I don't know how I could've gone that deep without the intensity of my circumstances. Normally, I would have turned away. Somehow, I would have moved away from that discomfort. I would play golf, read a book, or watch TV. But having to sit with my imminent death in that Zen monastery and having nowhere to go forced me into a deeper understanding. That made it real for me.

After facing some of my greatest fears, I finally took possession of my life. I took full responsibility for my physical, mental, and spiritual health. It's up to me.

This struggle has significantly improved my ability to network, build teams, seek help, get support, and be open to the world around me. Now I see the whole world as my potential support structure. I go and ask for what I need.

I don't take my life for granted anymore. I'm grateful for my health and my life.

I'm still going to die. Life is impermanent, after all. At best, I've delayed it. But if I can live a more fulfilling and connected life along the way, that's winning.

My life has been completely transformed. The only thing I'm not sure has changed are my food allergies.

From time to time, I continue to test foods to see if I'm still allergic. Cherries have always bothered me. Recently, my son got a bag of beautiful Bing cherries. I thought I would try one. I took one little bite. There was immediate swelling in my jaw and throat. I felt nauseated.

So there it was: No cherries.

Oh, well. *At least I can breathe again.*

12

Afterword: Reflections on The Journey

Unapologetic narcissism was essential at one point in this process. It was all about me because it had to be. I enjoyed that.

There's a part of me that has always loved being the center of attention. Being sick was an easy way to get there. It was a permission slip to make it all about myself without that being a problem.

By becoming healthy, I had lost the perfect excuse to not do anything I didn't want to do. Now I can't be the center of attention all the time.

That's probably for the best.

Now that I'm healthier, I'm expanding my worldview to include others again. I want to be of service to the world. My focus has shifted from me and my illness to other sufferers.

I am grateful for all the support, wisdom, and good fortune I was given in my darkest hours. I want to help other people who are in the dark place that I escaped. I want to share what has worked for me with whomever needs assistance.

Since recovering, I've talked to quite a few people who have respiratory issues. When I tell my story, many people bring me their stories about their loved ones' lungs breaking down.

Respiratory issues, like COPD and emphysema, are common and will become more common with the growing amount of pollution we have.

I want people who are suffering to know what I've learned and what is possible. With this book, I'm banging the drum and trying to bring attention.

Being a Good Steward

Throughout my journey, I gradually took on more responsibility. By sharing this message, I take huge responsibility to do it right. I want to be a good steward. I want to share, with integrity, what I've learned.

People who are suffering are in a vulnerable position. I do not want to be a snake-oil salesman. I want to offer a full range of possibilities without making unfounded promises of uncertain outcomes.

Underlying this process is uncertainty about what treatment or practice did what. I undertook a comprehensive program and had a great outcome, but I don't know precisely which variables were critical and which ones weren't. I can't pull things apart and point to specific results. I have only the whole package.

For example, most of the supplements I took were added all at once. It's worth noting that pulling any given result out of this is near impossible. There was no control group, no trial period. I took all of these things as a batch. For example, there wasn't a day where I took Detox Essentials but didn't take vitamin D.

I don't claim that following my path will provide the same

results.[21] I may have had a mild form of the disease. My body may respond to things that yours does not. Some factors listed here may have had no effect at all. I can't say. There is no control group for my life. Maybe it was a fluke. But I don't think so. Some parts might have been. But I could feel the difference directly with aspects like ingestion and nasal lavage.

I don't want to create the impression that "I know what will work for you." My goal is not to tell you what to do. The deeper truth I would want to convey is this: *You've got to make your own choices.* I'm simply sharing what has worked for me and what I've learned. Do with it whatever makes sense for you. This book is an encouragement to cut your own path — not to follow my path. With the conventional medical system, I was told there was just one path. But there isn't just one path.

What I Want to Pass Along

This is what I want to tell anyone suffering from bronchiectasis or another respiratory disease:

#1. Take 100% responsibility for your own health.

One of my espoused key values has always been to be 100% responsible for my life. I don't want to blame others or make excuses. Yet, I wasn't living that way. I wasn't living up to my own value system.

Also, part of me enjoys self-pity. It's a lot easier to just lie

---

[21] Both my brother and the author who wrote the anticancer book died of cancer while on the anticancer diet. Suzanne Friedman, the Zen priest with lung cancer, also died.

back, be passive, and feel sorry for myself rather than to fix things.

When I had full trust in the medical system, there was a luxury there: I didn't have to think deeply or for very long about my own body and what was happening. I had always laid the responsibility for my health on my doctors. I hadn't taken responsibility for things like daily exercise, sufficient sleep, being engaged with my diet, and watching and seeing how my body responded to stimuli. I hadn't paid attention. I allowed the doctor to hold all the information. I just showed up for my physicals. They charted the numbers and told me if I was in good shape or not. However, everyone needs to be their own medical concierge, so to speak, and to be in charge of their holistic health.

#2. Your body can heal itself. You can promote an environment and a lifestyle that helps the body do its best.

#3. Consider using my kit of specific tools, protocols, medicines, and techniques.

These are largely affordable and potentially beneficial for you. If you're suffering from respiratory ailments, I want to encourage you to try one, a few, or all of these things. I was surprised that some of these techniques were free/inexpensive and easy to do, such as Buteyko breathing, and yet I had never heard of them. In a lifetime of reading about asthma, they never came up. All these options were invisible. I hope to make them visible.

#4. Put together your own personalized strategy.

I encourage you to cut your own path and not just follow my own. View your situation as truly unique. Find out what works for you. Then take it where it needs to go.

I love bread, but I had to do what worked for me. And bread didn't work. If bread works for you, that's fine. But be alert to what works and doesn't work for you personally.

#5. Get clear.

So much of my success was the by-product of clarity. Victor Rothschild said, "Be cautious and bold." This means be cautious in making your plan and then bold in executing it. That's exactly what happened here. Clarity promoted boldness for me.

I appreciate the clarity that the doctors at Mayo gave me: "You are on your own. What we know to do, we have done. So if you do need more, you need to go figure it out." That was a gift.

When the initial diagnosis of bronchiectasis came, I was spinning with confusion and went into denial. I had no plan. I was lost and wondering, "What do I do?" The Zen retreat reduced that confusion and mind chatter.

First, I got clarity about how I was going to approach my life. Then I got clear on the idea of the medical concierge approach. Then I got clear about who I should listen to. I got clear ideas from them. I integrated everything into a clear approach. Then I followed it like a checklist. At each moment, it was clear what to do next.

A lot of the emotional upheaval that might have gone along with the whole process were already dealt with at the Zen retreat. By grieving everything, I was free to open and be fully into the adventure from that point forward.

With total clarity, I opened myself to this adventure.

#6. Set intentions.

Setting the intention of "complete respiratory restoration" was more important than I could have known. With that intention, I built a team to support me and developed a plan. Executing that plan is what saved me. I'm amazed how that bold but simple intention worked out.

#7. Make it boring.

One of my father's favorite maxims in investing was "vanilla is a pretty good flavor."

I made my approach boring. I took a lot of the drama out of it. I researched and met with experts to make my game plan. Without the protocol, there would've been more anxiety.

The success of this was tied to how boring it was. If it had been exciting and if I had been experimenting with new or truly risky techniques, it wouldn't have been good.

#8. If it has a high potential benefit, low cost, and no potential harm, try it.

I don't know if acupuncture had an effect at all. I couldn't really see the results, but I didn't see any harm, either.

Also, the breathing method has no credibility in conventional medicine (as far as I know). But it's free and harmless, so anyone with breathing problems should consider trying it for themselves. If it doesn't work, there's no cost or risk. But if it works, the benefits could be significant.

#9. Create a trustworthy system so you can act without doubt.

In retrospect, I eliminated a lot of dead ends by first building the team. I chose high-quality sources and then received high-quality recommendations. I learned credible techniques from credible sources. Because of this, the techniques I tried were more likely to be successful.

It was clear-cut from the beginning. It wasn't trial and error. We made the plan, and I trusted the plan. Then it was just a matter of implementing it.

Once I vetted an expert and trusted a process, I focused on running the program. Some things didn't have an immediate impact. Some things took months or years before I saw a difference. But I didn't constantly second-guess the plan.[22] I just measured the progress of that system along the way. Once the program was going, I was just a soldier.

#10. Overdoing defined every step of my journey.

My basic flaws are still there, but they're smaller now. I still overdo. I get excited about possibilities. I'm writing books, running a business, and have Zen retreats coming up. Who scheduled all this? Me. Even with taking care of myself, I am still trying to fit it all in. It will kill me if it's done to excess. Hopefully, I've learned enough of a lesson that I'm doing it short of excess. But let's be honest, my overdoing is also what saved me. My protocol had a certain element of excess

---

[22] This has parallels in my career as an investor.

and overdoing. There weren't half measures. Half measures wouldn't have done it.

#11. Even on successful journeys, success doesn't feel inevitable.

At the beginning, my journey didn't feel heroic. I felt desperate.

Success never felt certain going forward. The philosopher Søren Kierkegaard once said, "Life can only be understood backwards; but it must be lived forwards."

Not every journey ends in success. There was no guarantee that these things would have any impact. I could have tried all these things and stayed just as sick. I don't know how I would've handled that.

So realize that your despair and doubt are part of the process, and not an indicator of your future success.

#12. Don't expect a silver bullet or overnight success.

Even though — over the course of the entire journey — there was a huge, dramatic change, it happened gradually. No day was dramatically different from the day before. Even the Mayo news wasn't dramatic. It was an ongoing and gradual improvement, building on what had already been done.

There's a silver bullet mentality out there: "If I take this one thing, then everything will be better. Eat this one food and all of your problems will be solved. Take this one herb and everything will be cleared up." However, a holistic approach seems far more intelligent to me.

The silver bullet mentality misses out on all the possible options. If you change everything a little bit and create this organic approach, the body can heal itself. You're amiss if you're focused on doing just one thing. Look at the whole picture. The more you can develop a lifestyle that promotes the body's ability to heal itself, the less you're likely to suffer certain illnesses.

#13. Western medicine isn't a villain.

Western medicine may be seen as the villain to be defeated in this story. But it's not that way. The moral is not "forget Western medicine."

Villains have evil intent. I don't see anything malicious about that system. The allergist didn't do anything wrong. It's the system that's flawed. The conventional system can think only in conventional ways. It's blocked from any possibilities that fall outside that.

The villain was largely my own shadow — the one that did not take 100% responsibility for my life. I had let the conventional medical system call the shots. The mindset of "whatever conventional medical system says, that's what I'll do" needed to be defeated.

The moral is this: Use Western medicine first and take it as far as it serves you. Just don't sit on your hands when it can't take you where you need to go.

With the traditional system, I had reached the end of the road for my condition. I'm grateful that it took me as far as it did.

I still use conventional medicine. With my first glass of water in the morning, I still take omaprazole for stomach acid. I have acid reflux and it works, so I stick with it. I still have the Ventolin and the emergency stuff available if and when it's needed.

Also, conventional medicine is incorporating more and more

of the integrated approach. Mayo now has an acupuncture office. However, I don't know if nebulizing, which was such a home run for me, will ever get tested by the medical establishment.

Regardless, it's your body. You can't wait around for them to figure it out.

13

Appendix: My Daily Recovery Checklist

___ *64 oz. of water*
___ *5 servings of fruits & vegetables*
___ *30 minutes of cardio*
___ *5 meals per day:*
___ *Breakfast – fruit/protein/water*
___ *Snack – protein shake/water*
___ *Lunch – veggie/protein/water*
___ *Snack – protein shake/water*
___ *Dinner – veggie/protein/water*
___ *12 hours of sleep (8 hours minimum)*
___ *Supplements (morning)*
___ *Supplements (evening)*
___ *Nasal lavage (morning)*
___ *Nasal lavage (evening)*
___ *Breath flow meter*
___ *Nebulizer (morning)*
___ *Nebulizer (evening)*

Acknowledgements

I'm so very grateful for the support I got when I needed it.

An enormous thank you to Austin Pierce, my co-writer, and without whom this project would never have gotten off the ground. He saw the possibilities of this story of being an inspiration to others and cracked the whip on turning this idea into a finished product.

I'm grateful for my office team (Gayle Rupp and Shelby Pierce, and my partner, Corey Wrenn). They kept the business going and offered unquestioned support every step of the way.

Deep gratitude for Jun Po Roshi, his encouragement, and the insights that came to me at the Dai Bosatsu Zen Meditation Center. There I saw that I could go grasping and clinging (grieving) or dancing and singing (embracing life). That decision took me into the integrated world. What a choice. And then to have it all work out so well. What an amazing experience.

Great thanks to all the professionals at Mayo. While I may disagree with their worldview, I never doubted their excellence and commitment to the medicine they practice.

I'm grateful for my GP, Dr. Jung. I appreciated his support and open-mindedness to different healing modalities.

A huge thanks to my friend, David Lang, who reached out when I really needed it. He was my ticket into the naturopathic world and referred me to Dr. Daenell.

A gigantic thank you to Dr. Carrie-Louise Daenell whose

innovative naturopathic methods were so effective in my healing process. I especially appreciated her positive outlook and encouragement when I so needed it.

Big thanks to my acupuncturist, Jade, and her dedication to her craft of Chinese medicine.

I am so blessed to be a father. Thanks to my children, John, Charlie, and Danielle, who have helped me grow in a thousand ways. Hopefully, this book is a giving back to them, a reminder to take 100% responsibility for their health and their bodies.

Most of all, great love and thanks to my wife, Kay, my high school sweetheart and greatest teacher. She patiently waited for me to catch up with her on alternative healing modalities. Thanks, honey.

Made in the USA
San Bernardino, CA
24 March 2020